NRP Manual

Neonatal Resuscitation Program

Julie Johnson RN, MSN

NRP Manual

ISBN-13: 978-1502403452

ISBN-10: 1502403455

Printed in the United States of America.

Dedication

To all Pediatric Nurses

Neonatal resuscitation

Introduction

For the transition from intrauterine to extra-uterine life to be successful, certain physiologic adaptation ought to take place successfully in a neonate. Some changes take place long time after birth and must be necessitated by resuscitation. According Zaichkin, Kattwinkel & Weiner (2011), ninety percent of all infants' physiologic changes are successfully completed at delivery without requiring any special assistance. However, about nine percent of infants will need some intervention, and one percent will require extensive resuscitative measures at birth

Birth asphyxia causes most neonatal deaths. Birth asphyxia is defined as failure to initiate and sustain breathing at birth. The medical team conducting the delivery of the infant should be on the alert for an emergency tray to conduct the resuscitation whenever birth asphyxia happens. Resuscitation is a lifesaving procedure that if not conducted a high mortality rate of the infants will be recorded (McAdams, 2014). It is necessary that the resuscitation procedure be done on the correct way. Poor resuscitation procedure can complicate the already compromised respiratory system.

Recommendation on Basic Newborn Resuscitation

The degree of asphyxia differs from one newborn to another. Consequently, there are leading cues on how long the infant needs the resuscitation. Not all the newborns with asphyxia at birth have the same strength of recommendation for resuscitation. The leading cues that indicate extend of asphyxia are five (Gunay, 2013). These cues are checked on the newborn soon after birth. First, the midwife conducting delivery should assess the mother if she reached the expected date of delivery.

In the event that the baby is born pre-maturely then it is more likely than not that, the baby will need resuscitation. If the infant is born prematurely then resuscitation begins by delaying the cord clamping. The clamping of the cord should not be done earlier than one minute after birth. Delay in clamping the cord is to allow the exchange of oxygenated blood between the mother and the infant. Exceptions in delay of cord clamping is when the baby is a preterm infant and need positive airway ventilation on the resuscitation.

Second cue is when the infant delays to cry spontaneously immediately after birth. The first-line resuscitation procedure on such scenario calls for drying of the infant and stimulation by rubbing the back of the infant. The rubbing should be 2-3 times before clamping the cord. Then a positive airway ventilation should be initiated until the infant can breathe spontaneously. Most infants fail to cry immediately after birth (Gunay, 2013).

Third cue is when the infant is born in clear amniotic fluid. Most of the infants swallow the amniotic fluid and later compromise the respiratory system. Infants with amniotic fluids in the respiratory system should undergo suctioning of nostril first then proceed to the mouth. Care need to be taken when suctioning the mouth since it can stimulate vagal nerve complicate the asphyxia. Suctioning of the upper respiratory system and mouth is to make the respiratory system patent. Consequently, the infant will be able to breath freely without obstructions by amniotic fluids (Gunay, 2013). In the effect, the cardiopulmonary resuscitation can proceed after ensuring the airway is patent. The compression and mechanical ventilation can be done unless all the fluids are removed

The fourth cue that could be consequential to infant resuscitation is an infant born in meconium-stained amniotic fluid. The strength of recommendation for resuscitation is very strong on this scenario. However, the intrapartum suctioning of the mouth and nose of the infant is not recommended. In case the suctioning is done, the baby may delay to be delivered resulting in more compromised respiratory problems.

The fifth cue is an exception for the baby born in meconium stained amniotic fluid but initiate spontaneous breathing. In such scenario, the tracheal suctioning is not recommended. Spontaneous breathing is indicative of adequate respiratory efforts and the airway is patent. The infant will free the amniotic fluid by coughs and crying. However, tracheal suctioning should be done to the infants born in meconium stained amniotic fluid and cannot initiate spontaneous breathing. Positive pressure ventilation should be next performing the suctioning.

Performing the Resuscitation

ABC is very essential. One need to ensure the airway is patent, and then breathing and circulatory system of the neonate (Rovamo, 2013).

Prevention of Hypothermia

The infant should be dried after birth to prevent heat loss. The fluid on the body of the neonate accelerates the rate of heat loss. In case heat is lost profoundly, the neonate is likely to have a compromised breathing. Consequently, impaired respiratory system will necessitate resuscitation of the neonate. Then 100% oxygen should be given for assisted ventilation. In case the supplemental oxygen is not available then, positive pressure ventilation is initiated with the normal room air. Oxygenation is very necessary as it boost the partial pressure of oxygen. As a result, the tissues that poorly supplied with oxygen will be oxygenated. The characteristic blue coloration that is indicative of low oxygen supply will disappear once oxygenation is adequate. Most cases a laryngeal mask airway is effective, as an alternative for establishing an airway if bag-mask ventilation is ineffective and intubation has failed (Rovamo, 2013).

Suctioning

Suctioning should be done with a lot of care. It should be aseptic procedure when suctioning the nostrils for any fluids. Orally ought not to be aseptic. The suctioning should be done from inside outside in a circular manner for it to be effective. Care need to be taken when doing the suctioning as the neonate can be bruised with the tube. A proper size suctioning tube should be used since large one tends to compromise the intra suctioning period.

The large suctioning tube of the neonate becomes obstructive and abrasive on the membranes. Such tubes can result in bleeding and obstructive apnea that can cause death. Such occurrence happens because of exacerbation of apnea in neonate with severe asphyxia. The order of suctioning begins with the nose then proceeds to the mouth, which ought not to be aseptic.

Chest compression

Chest compression should be administered in case the heart rate is absent or below 60 beats per minute even after adequate ventilation for thirty seconds. The two thumb that encircles the neonate should be used in the chest compression. The depth of compression should be considered because forceful compression can injure the fragile sternum. The depth of compression should be a third the anterior-posterior diameter of the chest and sufficient to generate a palpable pulse. The compressions are alternated with mechanical ventilation until spontaneous breathing is observed. The ratio of compression to bagging the neonate should be 30: 1. The thirty compression should be proceeded by bagging via facemask. In doing the compression, the muscles are put into metabolic activity. Metabolic activity results in accumulation waste products, which ought to be removed by enhancing oxygenation. Without alternating with bagging, the neonate can complicate.

Medication

Neonates on resuscitation need some resuscitative drugs to help them pick faster (Trevisanuto, 2005). For the effectiveness of the chest compressions and mechanical ventilation using an amp bag, emergency medication should be added. Such medication is mostly for volume expansion and vascular access. An example of such essential resuscitative drug is epinephrine. Epinephrine should be given when the heart rate is below 60 beat per minutes after a minimum of thirty seconds of chest compression. Epinephrine ensures that the cardiac system correspond to the resuscitative measure taken such as chest compression and bagging via the facial mask. A mismatch between airway intervention such as oxygenation and blood circulatory system reduces the effectiveness resuscitation effort.

Discontinuation of Resuscitation

The resuscitation team should understand when to stop resuscitation. Sometimes stopping resuscitation may be beneficial than doing it continuously. In case after the long resuscitation and the breathing remain uninitiated then it is appropriate to stop resuscitation. Circumstances such as low birth weight and gestational age anomalies increase non-responsiveness to intervention. Such neonates who fail to respond should be taken to extensive resuscitative measure.

Pediatric Assessment (level of consciousness, breathing, color)

Precise assessment of a child with an acute illness or suffering from an injury requires certain crucial knowledge and skills. Most of the children presenting in the ER often have a mild, moderate illness and injury and stay alert. In the assessment of these patients' illnesses and injuries, several methodologies and severity scales can be incorporated for assessing the levels of consciousness. However, these methodologies often lack accuracy, especially when it comes to infants and toddlers (Donnelly, 2009). This implies that although the methods will help in classifying the moderate to critically ill or injured child, it will however not help in the recognition of crucial signs that help in noting the early symptoms of system strain in the sick or wounded child who is still operating well or looks well. A nurse needs to apply critical thinking in assessing pediatrics as their shift from consciousness to unconsciousness is very rapid.

1. **Evaluation-primary assessment, secondary assessment, diagnostic tests**

Diagnostic tests refer to any test that is used to determine the existence of an illness or disease. For example, there are cases where the test is carried out in order to fully diagnose someone or to affirm that a patient is free of any disease. Diagnostic tests include CT scans, bronchoscopy, x-rays, oesophageal ultrasound and angiography.

The main aim of carrying out primary assessment is to immediately identify life threatening problems. The primary assessment mainly aims at stabilizing the patient, identify life-threatening conditions in the patient in order of risk and initiate for treatment immediately. Secondary assessment will come after the primary assessment has been fully carried out and the patient's vital signs have all been assessed. It comprises of checking the patient history and physical examination of the patient.

2. Respiratory Assessment, Circulatory Assessment

Respiratory assessment consists of four main components, which include inspection, palpation, percussion and auscultation. Inspection involves the medical practitioner using their eyes and ears to assess a varying number of things about their patients. Some of the main things that should be observed include pursed lip breathing, noisy breathing, skin color, coughing, respiratory rate, patterns, and chest wall abnormalities.

In the palpation phase, the healthcare personnel uses their fingers and hands during the physical examination. They will touch and feel the patient's body in order to determine the consistency, size, texture, tenderness and location of a body organ or body part. Percussion on the other hand involves the technique of tapping body hands by using the fingers and certain instruments during the physical examination. It is often used to determine the presence or absence of fluids in certain body organs and the borders, size and consistency of body organs (Baren, 2008).

Percussion of a body organ normally produces a certain sound that will in turn indicate the presence of a certain tissue within that particular body part or organ. Lastly, there is auscultation. During auscultation, the patient is supposed to sit upright while taking in deep breaths through the mouth. Any outside noise should be eliminated if possible. The examiner will then listen to the sounds arising within the body organs.

While assessing circulation, the medical practitioner should determine whether the child has a pulse or is in shock. One should keep in mind that children and infants are only capable of tolerating only small amounts of blood loss before they suffer circulatory compromise. It is important to assess and control any bleeding early in the circulatory assessment. Circulatory assessment should not only focus on the circulatory status but also try to correct any inadequate circulation to other body organs of the infant or child. The main measures of circulatory assessment are heart rate and blood pressure. However, changes in the skin percussion can be used as indicators of compensated shock.

Types of shock: (Hypovolemic, distributive, cardiogenic, obstructive)

a. Cardiogenic Shock

In cardiogenic shock, the forward flow of blood is often inadequate due to a defect in the cardiac function. It normally happens when the heart cannot properly pump blood through the body system. This could be due to impairment caused to the heart from myocardial infarction that results in enough damage to the heart to impair its proper functioning. Furthermore, a disease or virus could also be a cause of cardiogenic shock.

b. Hypovolemic Shock

Hypo simply means lack of or low, while volemic refers to fluid volume. In an instance when a patient is injured and profusely bleeding, the volume of blood that the body is able to deliver reduces substantially resulting to the patient experiencing hypovolemic shock. This kind of shock is quite common in patients who have suffered from trauma and have external bleeding. However, a patient can equally suffer from internal bleeding from an illness or injury, which can quickly result in the patient falling into a hypovolemic shock state.

c. *Distributive Shock*

Distributive shock occurs when the intravascular volume is markedly abnormal due to a decrease in vascular resistance, such as it happens to occur in fainting where blood pools in the venous instead of the arterial portion of the blood flow.

Cardiac output may be augmented, normal or small in patients who experience distributive shock. Several causes may cause distributive shock such as septic shock, neurogenic shock, anaphylactic shock and acute adrenal insufficiency. However, there are drugs that result in vasodilation thus resulting in the patient experiencing distributive shock (Baren, 2008).

d. *Obstructive Shock*

The main characteristic of obstructive shock is the impedance of sufficient cardiac filling of the ventricles leading to a significant decrease in the cardiac output. As the distribution of blood decreases, the patients' tissues may begin to die because of lack of oxygen and necessary nutrients. There are certain patients who have a high risk of suffering from obstructive shock such as those on bed rest and those who have mobility issues and do not move around so much. Furthermore, patients with chest injuries have a higher risk of suffering from obstructive shock.

Diagnostic tests: Arterial blood gas

Arterial blood gas is the measurement of the oxygen level in the blood flowing through the arteries. The process normally involves puncturing an artery with a thin needle and drawing a small amount blood from the artery. The most commonly chosen puncture for this process is the radial artery.

The main reason for carrying out this test is in order to determine the blood pH level, the part pressure of carbon dioxide and oxygen and the level of bicarbonate in the blood. In addition, there are instances where the test determines the lactate level. However, the required sample to carry out the arterial blood gas test may be difficult to acquire because of the diminished pulses in some patients and constant patient movement (King, 2008).

Diminished pulses may be a reflection of low blood pressure or poor peripheral circulation in the patient as a result of the illness. The constant movement is due to the pain that comes as a result of the arterial puncture. In an infant who weighs less than 30 pounds, arterial blood can be obtained from the capillary stick instead, and in the case of a newborn, it is obtained from the umbilical catheter. Although arterial puncture is a skill that can easily be learned, there may be instances where certain complications may come about as a result. Such complications include trauma and occlusion, infection, vessel spasm and embolization. However, in a case where a skilled practitioner performs arterial puncture, it offers safe and reliable information, which is useful in patient management.

Venous Blood Gas

Venous blood gas (VBG) is a substitute method used in the measurement or estimation of carbon dioxide and pH in the blood that does not require arterial puncture.

VBG is most preferred as compared to ABG, particularly for patients in the intensive care unit given that they already have a central venous catheter from which the venous blood can easily be obtained.

The VBG test is useful in assessing oxygen and carbon dioxide gas exchange, respiratory functions such as hypoxia and acid/base balance in the patients. Furthermore, it can also be incorporated in the evaluation of asthma, chronic obstructive pulmonary disease and various types of lung disease such as coronary artery disease. Abnormal results of the VBG tests may be due to metabolic, lung and kidney diseases. However, patients who may have a history of head or neck injuries will also likely have abnormal VBG results (Donnelly, 2009)

Hemoglobin and Hematocrit

Both the hemoglobin and the hematocrit refer to specific characteristics of the red blood cells, but they however measure different things. The hemoglobin is a compound in the red blood cells that transports oxygen to other cells in the body. The hemoglobin tests measures how much hemoglobin is present in the blood. The test is often carried out when doctors want to determine the patient's general health and patients' blood chemistry. The hematocrit test on the other hand is carried out to determine the total percentage of the volume of the blood that contains the red blood cells. The measurement will be dependent on the number of the red blood cells and the size of the red blood cells.

Central venous pressure monitoring

The central venous pressure (CVP) is the direct measurement of blood pressure in the central veins adjacent to the heart. It shows the average right atrial pressure and are most of the times used to estimate the right ventricular preload. Although the CVP does not measure the blood volume directly, it may however be used from time to time. In CVP monitoring, a catheter is inserted through a vein and advanced until the tip lies in or on the right atrium. Given the fact that there are no valves present between the junction of the vena cava and the right atrium, the pressure reading at the end of the diastole directly transfers to the catheter. CVP monitoring is important because it gives the necessary information pertaining to the body's blood volume or fluid status and the right ventricular function.

CVP can be monitored intermittently or continuously. There are three main approaches used in the measuring of the pressure in the right atrium. One would be using a water manometer attached to the attached to the CV catheter. Second would be using a line placed directly into the right atrium which is then attached to the transducer system. Lastly, would be using a proximal lumen of a pulmonary artery catheter.

The normal CVP ranges from 5 to 10 cm H_2O. A number of underlying conditions that may alter venous return, flowing blood volume or cardiac activity may in turn impact on the CVP. For instance, if the circulating blood was to increase due to increase in venous return to the heart, the CVP is most likely to rise. On the other hand, if the flowing volume decreases, the CVP will drop. Overdistention or underfilling of the venous collecting system can easily be identified by monitoring the CVP before the clinical symptoms become apparent. The CVP can be measures in instances where the patients with hypertension are not responding to the basic clinical management implemented, or in patients requiring infusions or inotropes, or in patients who seem to be experiencing continuing hypervolemia secondary to major fluid loss or shifts (Parthasarathy, 2013).

Invasive Arterial pressure monitoring

Invasive blood pressure (IBP) monitoring is a commonly employed method in the Intensive Care Unit (ICU) and in the operating room. It entails the insertion of a catheter into a suitable artery and displaying the recorded pressure wave on the monitor. Patients who are undergoing invasive blood pressure monitoring should be under close supervision constantly given that they may likely suffer blood loss in any case the line comes off. The method is often reserved for critically ill patients who are likely to experience rapid changes in their blood pressure.

Normal or acceptable blood pressure varies from one patient to another depending on the patient's age, health status and clinical information. At birth, the expected blood pressure is normally 80 mmHg. This number rises steadily through childhood, such that in a young adult the expected blood pressure is 100/80 mmHg. In order to determine whether the recorded reading is normal for that particular patient, it shall be compared to the "normal" for that patient. In the incorporation of this technique in blood measurement, the cannula is place into an artery (normally radial, dorsalis pedis or brachial). The cannula will then be connected to a sterile system filled with fluid which is then connected to an electronic patient monitor. The main benefit of this method is that the pressure is measured beat-by-beat and the waveform easily readable and displayed for monitoring.

Chest x-ray, echocardiogram, peak expiratory flow rate

Peak flow rate is a simple, quantitative, reproducible measurement of the existence and severity of air flow obstruction. It is an important tool often used in the monitoring, exacerbations and daily long term monitoring. Peak expiratory flow (PEF) can be measured by the use of Mini Wright peak flow meters which are inexpensive and affordable to many. PEF is a quick and easy way for health care practitioners to measure and record predicted normal PEF values, while taking into consideration the height and age of the child as a point of reference.

However, the value which is considered "normal" is of a rather wide range and hence the test is dependent on the effort of the pediatrician. Health care practitioners can easily teach their patients to carry the PEF test on their own given the easy nature of the method.

Respiratory distress and failure

Respiratory distress is a state of increased work of breathing, while respiratory failure is a state inadequate oxygenation or ventilation. Respiratory failure may or may not be preceded by respiratory failure. Assessment of an infant's respiratory status often begins with the Pediatric Assessment Triangle. Infants and children often have unique clinical condition that may result in respiratory problems. Respiratory distress is a form of respiratory failure that comes about as a result of varying disorders that may cause fluid to accumulate in the lungs and low oxygen levels in the blood. According to research, quick identification of respiratory distress in in the pediatric patient is crucial before it escalates into respiratory failure.

The main symptoms of respiratory failure often manifest themselves in the patient 24 to 48 hours after injury, but may take up to 5 days to be notable in the patient. The patient is likely to have shortness of breath, and usually shallow and rapid breathing. Crackling or wheezing sounds can be heard when the pediatrician auscultates the lungs. The small oxygen availability in the blood will also cause the child's skin to be cyanotic.

Conversely, respiratory failure is a situation in which one or all the gas exchange functions fails i.e. oxygenation and carbon dioxide elimination. The situation can either be acute or chronic. It is safe to construe that this condition will likely occur in a patient whose respiratory distress was not handled properly. The main difference between respiratory distress and respiratory failure is that in respiratory distress the patent is still breathing, while in respiratory failure the patient stops breathing completely (Taussig, 2008). Respiratory failure normally occurs when the patients' lungs are incapable of properly removing carbon dioxide from the infant's blood. This will in turn result in too much accumulation of carbon dioxide in the system which will harm the patient's body organs. There are certain illnesses that that affect infants breathing that will result in respiratory failure such as chronic obstructive pulmonary disease (prevents air from properly flowing in and out of the system) and spinal cord injuries (may damage nerves that control breathing).

Management of upper respiratory airway obstruction

The most shared cause of upper respiratory obstruction is the tongue. The management of a patient with upper respiratory obstruction will vary depending on the cause of the obstruction, the level of skill and competence of the rescuer, and the availability of aids to perform the necessary airway techniques.

Obstruction of the upper airway is a life threatening condition that if not properly managed may possibly result in the patient's death. The main aim is to secure the patient from getting a heart attack or possibly suffering irreversible brain damage that can take place within minutes of the airway obstruction..

Management of Lower respiratory Airway obstruction.

Lower respiratory airway obstruction normally results from the infection or irritation from certain particular particles or substances. It normally occurs between the larynx and the narrow passages of the lungs. The main symptoms include air trapping, an increased AP diameter and barrel chest. The common simple ways of helping a patient with lower airway obstruction include chin lift, jaw thrust and performing adjuncts.

Intraosseous access.

In a critical resuscitation circumstance, after the airway has been secured and adequate breathing and gas exchange fully established back to normal, the next priority should be to obtain vascular access. Most of the times, this is difficult to attain especially in children and infants. The physiologic progressions of shock and hypothermia with subsequent vascular tightening which are normally notable in the resuscitative state may later on complicate the issue of venous access and make it worse.

In addition, the expertise of most healthcare personnel when it comes to attending to children widely varies.

Instraosseous access has been used for years and is considered safe, reliable and can easily used by medical practitioners who are not highly skilled when it comes to handling children as a way of introducing blood products, colloids, medications and crystalloids into the regular circulation (Parthasarathy, 2013) .

References

Baren, J. M. (2008). *Pediatric emergency medicine*. Philadelphia: Saunders/Elsevier.

Donnelly, L. F. (2009). *Fundamentals of pediatric radiology*. Philadelphia: Saunders.

Parthasarathy, A. (2013). *Partha's fundamentals of pediatrics*. New Delhi: Jaypee Brothers
   Publishers.

King, C., & Henretig, F. M. (2008). *Textbook of pediatric emergency procedures*.

Philadelphia: Wolters Kluwer Health/Lippincott Williams & Wilkins.

Gunay, I., Agin, H., Devrim, I., Apa, H., Tezel, B., & Ozbas, S. (2013). Resuscitation
skills of   pediatric residents and effects of Neonatal Resuscitation Program training.
Pediatrics   International, 55(4), 477-480. doi:10.1111/ped.12081

McAdams, R., McPherson, R., Batra, M., & Gerelmaa, Z. (2014). Characterization of
Health Care Provider Attitudes Toward Parental Involvement in Neonatal Resuscitation-
Related   Decision Making in Mongolia. *Maternal & Child Health Journal, 18*(4), 920-
929.   doi:10.1007/s10995-013-1319-5

Rovamo, L. M., Mattila, M., Andersson, S., & Rosenberg, P. H. (2013). Testing of
midwife   neonatal resuscitation skills with a simulator manikin in a low-risk delivery
unit. *Pediatrics   International, 55*(4), 465-471. doi:10.1111/ped.12083

Taussig, L. M., Landau, L. I., & Le, S. P. N. (2008). *Pediatric respiratory medicine*.
   Philadelphia: Mosby/Elsevier.

Trevisanuto, D., Ferrarese, P., Cavicchioli, P., Fasson, A., Zanardo, V., & Zacchello, F. (2005). Knowledge gained by pediatric residents after neonatal resuscitation program courses. *Pediatric Anesthesia*, *15*(11), 944-947. doi:10.1111/j.1460-9592.2005.01589.x

Zaichkin, J., Kattwinkel, J., Weiner, G. M., American Heart Association., & American Academy of Pediatrics. (2011). Instructor manual for neonatal resuscitation. Elk Grove Village, IL: American Heart Association.

Have you bought this book by the same author?

www.amazon.com

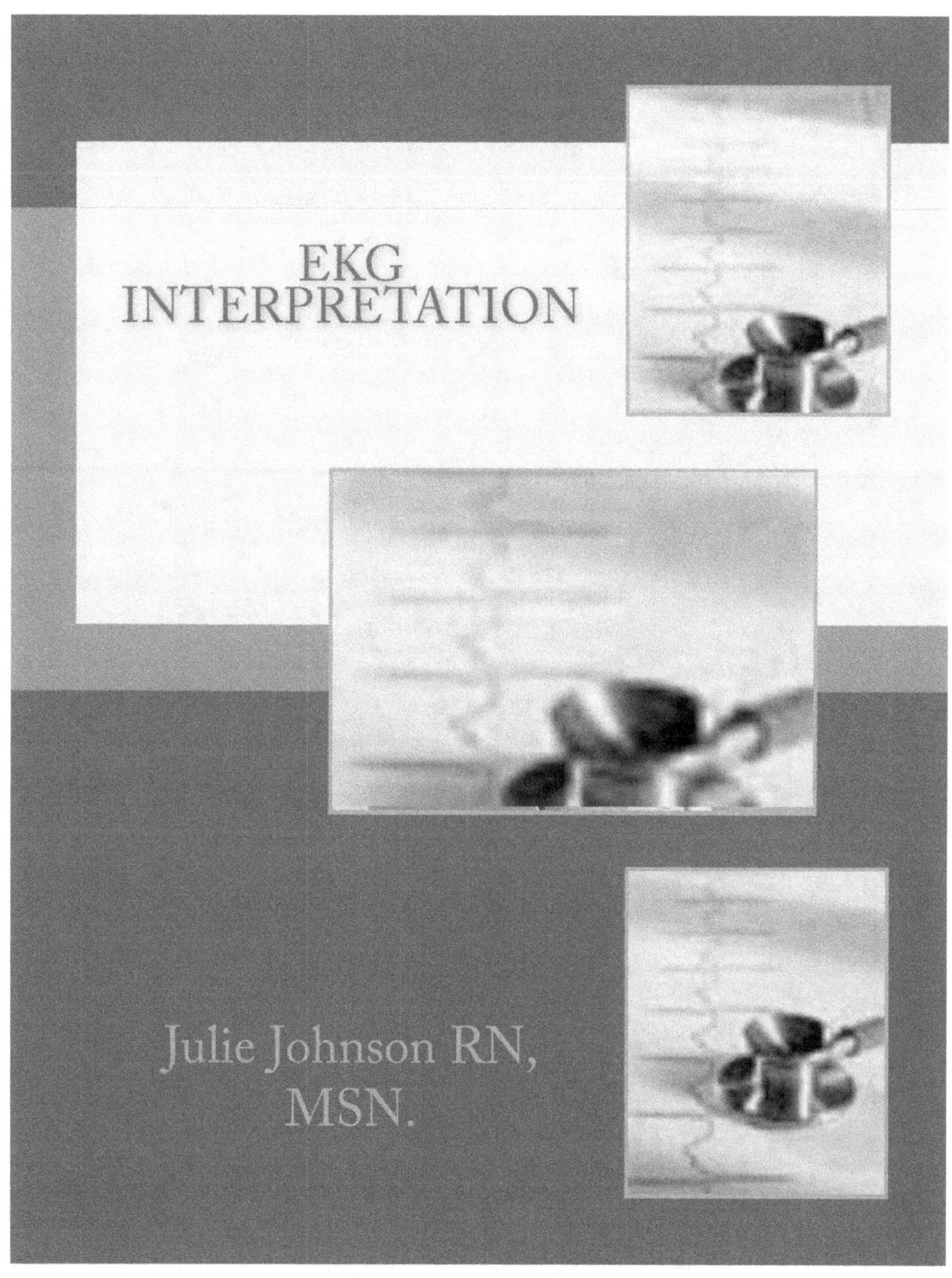

www.ingramcontent.com/pod-product-compliance
Lightning Source LLC
Chambersburg PA
CBHW081249170526

45165CB00009B/3255